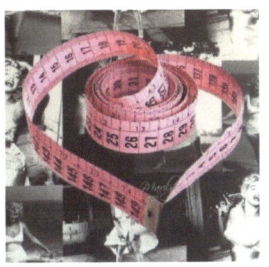

This book belongs to you,
the beautiful

who got her copy on

This is your book to document your journey on
Your Wardrobe Diet

The Wardrobe Diet

Buy less, wear more, always look and feel fabulous
by
Gay Richardson

Founder of Style Me Confident and creator of The Wardrobe Diet

Dedication

This book is dedicated to my dear departed Mum, my Dad and my adored daughters. To my Mum for her radical thinking, her glamorous style and her healthy attitude to life. By default, as she only lived until she was 47, she gave me a hugely compelling reason to be obsessively healthy so I could see my daughters and their children grow up.

To my Dad for always being encouraging and telling me to 'flash your smile!' To my dearest daughters, Jessie-Jan and Paris-Lily, for their endless patience with my technical skills, footwear and for making me laugh.

Contents

Introduction

Hello Beautiful!

Thank you for buying this book, I really hope that you enjoy it.

I wanted to explain how you can learn to love and accept the body you have and know what clothes to buy to motivate you to maintain the size you want to be and so enjoy getting dressed every day!

Before we start here's a bit about me and how The Wardrobe Diet came about.

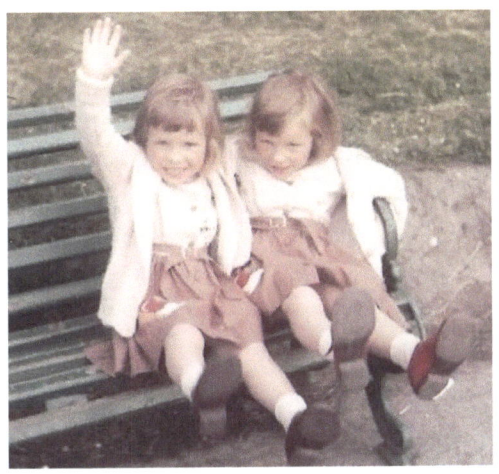

Since a very early age I have understood the power of clothes and how they make you feel. My first realisation was when I was age 4 ½ and my dad bought me a dress with appliqued vegetables in bright colours on it and I remember absolutely loving it, as it made me feel so happy, every time I wore it.

My other realisation was the importance of a healthy lifestyle (having lost my dear Mum to cancer when I was almost 21).
Initially I had wanted to be a dietician, but a spectacular fail at 'O' level chemistry prevented that career. However, I still remained fascinated by foods and did my BSc (Hons) in Food Marketing Sciences.

Over the next twenty years I had careers in events management and educational sales - nothing to do with clothes or keeping healthy, but always helping people.

My two beautiful daughters have always inspired and motivated me to keep healthy so that I would be there for them, all of their lives, and for any future grandchildren!

During those years, my love of clothes never waned and wherever I went I was known as the queen of mixing and matching because I created different outfits from the clothes that were already in my wardrobe.

In 2004 I had a bit of a 'career crisis' and I distinctly remember sitting at home wondering what on earth I could do next. I wanted to do something that could combine helping others and make me feel valued and happy too.

After watching one of Trinny and Susannah's hit UK TV shows 'What Not to Wear', I realized that I would love to inspire women to learn to love their bodies through the art of dressing.
I was fascinated to see how easily clothes can transform women's opinion of themselves, helping them to feel inspired, happier, and more confident, often for the first time in years.

This reminded me of my younger self's conviction that clothes have the power to transform how you feel about yourself.

Boom! That was it!

Ever since that moment I have been passionately convinced that I can make a difference to how you feel about yourself by teaching you what style and colours of clothes to wear.

So in 2005, I started Style Me Confident.

I did my training at the London College of Fashion where I learnt the technical and intricate details of styling, which answered the 'why' certain styles did or didn't work for me and consequently, for you too.

The gift of confidence through clothes – so simple!

I have been featured and worked with a number of national and local companies and publications including O2, Champneys, M&S Bank and The Mail on Sunday 'You' Magazine.

I won the 'Woman In Fashion' award at the Sussex Woman of the Year Awards, in 2013.

I have worked on a one-to-one basis with hundreds of women just like you, ranging from age 14-80 and sizes 6-24, through Style Me Confident and in my role as Debenhams resident Personal Shopper.

I always strive to bring happiness and relief to women, in a kind and sensitive way, inspiring them to love themselves, celebrate their beauty, and feel confident and happy about the way they look through what they wear… and always with a sense of fun!

I've never used scales to monitor my weight, I've always used my clothes as a guide. I've strived to stay the same weight as I **love** my clothes and I've invested a lot of time, effort and money in building up a collection of great pieces that are perfect for me, so I always want them to fit.

My wardrobe of clothes motivates me to eat healthily and exercise to maintain the same size and so combining my two passions - how clothes make you feel and living a healthy lifestyle. I update with accessories, footwear and a few key pieces each season.

The name 'The Wardrobe Diet™' came as the result of my eureka moment in late 2015.

I was talking to my business partner about writing a blog about how my wardrobe works for me and I suddenly realised that my 'way of living' was the essence of The Wardrobe Diet™. It's also what I have been teaching my clients for the past 11 years, but now it had a name.

My mission is to share this 'diet' and way of living with as many women as possible, in my lifetime. So I've put The Wardrobe Diet™ online **www.thewardrobediet.co.uk**

This book explains the concept and benefits of The Wardrobe Diet. Then you can choose to either take advantage of our extra special offer to you – at the end- or learn from any personal stylist.

I hope that it will inspire you as much as it inspires me.

Chapter 1:
The wardrobe's full …
yet I've 'nothing to wear'?

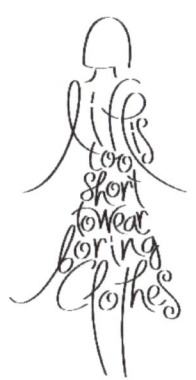

'I had always struggled with what to wear and felt dowdy, inferior, out of place and conscious of what I was wearing. Since working with Gay my confidence has soared, I feel gorgeous. People say 'you always look fabulous.'

Lucy, working Yummy Mummy, Selsey

There are not many things you have to do every day, but certainly one of them is getting dressed!

You can use your clothes to make you feel confident at the beginning of every single day.

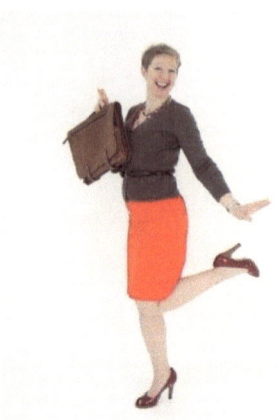

It is unlikely that you have been taught 'how to dress' even though it's a fundamental life skill.

Generally, you know the basics, but are maybe unsure what styles flatter your shape, what fabrics to choose, what colours to select to make you look radiant or how to combine pieces to make efficient use of your wardrobe.

You could be anyone of these women:

- a modern-day superwoman - continually multitasking;
- a yummy mummy - works part-time, juggling too many balls;
- a professional lady - who needs to dress to impress and always feel confident ;
- a nifty fifty-year-old - too young to wear twin sets, too old for leggings;
- a gorgeous grandma - recently retired, still raring to go!

Whichever you are, I can assure you that we all have similar issues.

Here's a list of the top eight most common ones - just tick which apply to you…go on, be honest (no-one will see this, except you.)

Top 8 Common Issues:

1. You dislike parts of your body, because they make you feel really self-conscious; ☐

2. You're fed up with always wearing the same sort of clothes; ☐

3. You have far too many clothes ; ☐

4. You want to maintain one size; ☐

5. You get frustrated or depressed by clothes shopping as you can't find what you like or what fits; ☐

6. You often just wear what you wore the day before, keeping nice clothes for best; ☐

7. You have a fail-safe go to 'uniform' that is comfortable, you don't feel self-conscious, yet you know it's not exciting; ☐

8. You want to look younger, yet still dress appropriately. ☐

Happiness is having an inner confidence that you radiate because you have accepted who you are, disguised the bits you don't like and are 'rocking' the parts you love, so you feel content and happy.

Over the past decade, I have discovered my clients are all different combinations of size, shape, colouring and every time I am fascinated by how unique you all are.

Yet you all have one thing in common and that's the beauty blind spot.

You are almost always blinkered and blind to your own beauty and uniqueness and loving the body you have. Instead you focus on the bits you dislike e.g. thighs/tummy/legs etc. and miss the whole fabulousness of yourselves.

You can be taught to dress with styles that flatter your shape so you can see the fabulousness of yourselves that's previously gone undiscovered!

You choose…

The *Vicious Circle*

You get up, you have 'nothing to wear', your clothes don't fit. So every morning you put the same thing on and start your day feeling blah. It undermines your confidence.

You eat comfort food as you feel unhappy, you are then tired so you don't exercise. Your sleep patterns may suffer. Then you wake up in the morning and it all starts again. Nooooooooooooooooooooooo!

or…

The Virtuous Circle

You always have something to wear, your clothes make you feel good, you get compliments. So you feel confident.

Because you feel good you feel like eating more healthily, then you have more energy, so you do exercise which makes you feel great.

This inspires you to keep up the healthy eating/exercise routines so you stay the same size, then your clothes always fit - the ones that make you look great. You'll probably sleep better. When you wake up you're happy and off you go again!

By moving from the vicious to the virtuous circle, it allows you to have a more positive effect on the people who are closest to you...your children, partner/husband, friends and most importantly, *yourself*.

Treat yourself with love, kindness, respect and appreciation every day and see how much better you will feel and the knock on effect on others around you.

So let's do 'Your Body Audit' and see how you feel about yourself, now.

Please answer the following questions as honestly as possible - only you will see it and then continue reading!

The Wardrobe Diet: Your Body Audit

Find a full length mirror and please look at yourself.
Please try to smile lovingly (not grimace!) and be kind.

What parts of you don't you like and why?

1.

2.

3.

(We are sticking at 3 here as we know you could go on forever but that's not helpful!)

Which parts do you like?
(Put at least 3- this could be more difficult, but keep smiling lovingly at yourself and you'll find them!)

1.

2.

3.

How tall are you?

Bra size

Shoe size

Shop size you mostly buy on top

Shop Size you mostly buy on bottom

Ask 2-3 people what are you best features
Write here and don't argue with them, just say "Thank you!"

What one piece of advice would you give your younger self today?

The Wardrobe Diet

Chapter 2:
How do you solve your
dressing dilemmas?

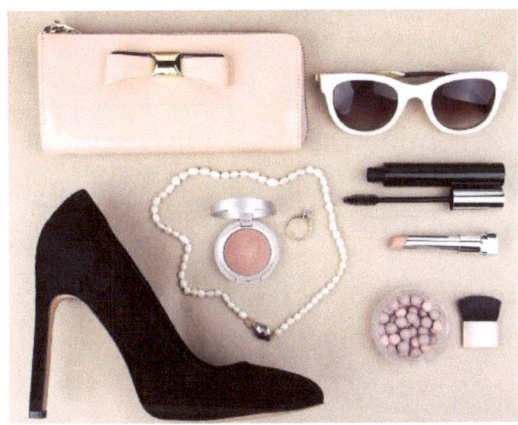

'I am very much enjoying having a wardrobe of clothes that I can wear, rather than what it was - 'a wardrobe of clothes and nothing to wear'. It certainly has made me more confident. Thank you.'

Ruth, professional business owner, mother with older sons

The Wardrobe Diet programme is a completely 'outside the box', different way of 'dieting'.

The word 'diet' actually comes from an ancient Greek word, meaning 'mode of living' and this is the essence of The Wardrobe Diet - live a happy life, motivated by the clothes in your wardrobe that you love, because they all fit, flatter and make you feel wonderful and confident.

Your clothes empower you to maintain the same size, with a combination of what you eat, the exercise you do, your mindset, and self-care – all of which affect your self-confidence and self-esteem.

It's all about accepting the body shape you have and learning to dress it in the most flattering way with the styles and colours that we teach you to choose.

You can learn styling tips that will instantly transform how you look and feel about yourself.

'I am having great fun trying out new ideas and have bought some new styles as suggested and they do make a difference, it's amazing. Have cleared out old colours that really don't suit, I wondered why I never felt quite right in them, now I know why!'

Sue, 60+, High Salvington

It's your clothes that will motivate you to stay the same size.

What you learn empowers you to throw away your scales and tape measure. Let your clothes guide you, so that you can still have cake, or anything else you enjoy - crisps, cheese, wine - but in moderation, so your clothes will always fit.

It's like learning any new skill e.g. cooking:

- you start with the basic 'recipe' and follow those steps;

- you stick to the tried and tested methods;

- you get great results;

- as you become more confident, you experiment with the 'ingredients', spicing it up or down, dependent on how you feel.

- You feel accomplished as you produce great food that has your 'take' on it

There are four steps that enable success:

Step 1 – learning your clever colours

Step 2 – understanding your beautiful body shape

Step 3 – re-organising your wonderful wardrobe

Step 4 – strategies for your successful shopping

What Step 1 – Your Clever Colours entails

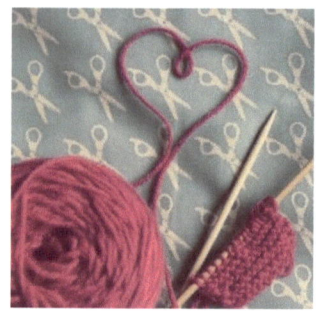

What colours suit you and why it's important to wear them.

Wearing your ideal colours will make you:

- look younger;

- look healthier;

- glow and

- feel happier and more confident.

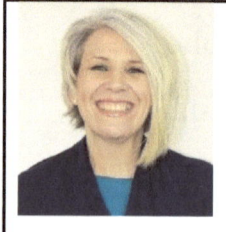 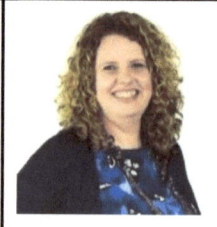 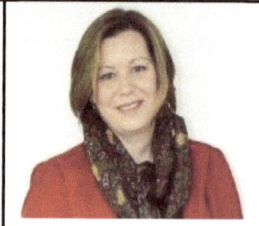 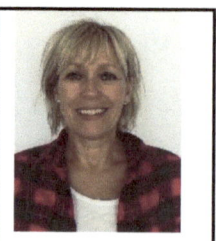

Knowing your ideal colours makes your shopping simple, successful and fun as you narrow down the choice by only buying colours that suit you.

It enables you to mix and match items, thus getting maximium wear out of everything in your wardrobe.

We use the popular seasonal colouring system - Autumn, Winter, Spring or Summer.

Your clever colours are determined by a combination of your skin tone, hair and eye colour.

Everyone has certain colour qualities and that's how we determine your clever colours. It works everytime !

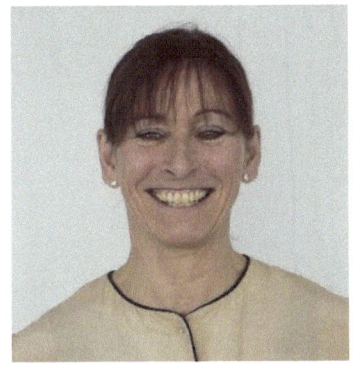

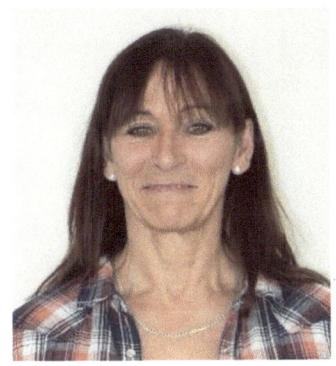

This colour is too pale.   These colours look great.

As part of our programme you have the choice to either print off your clever colours as a pdf (see below),

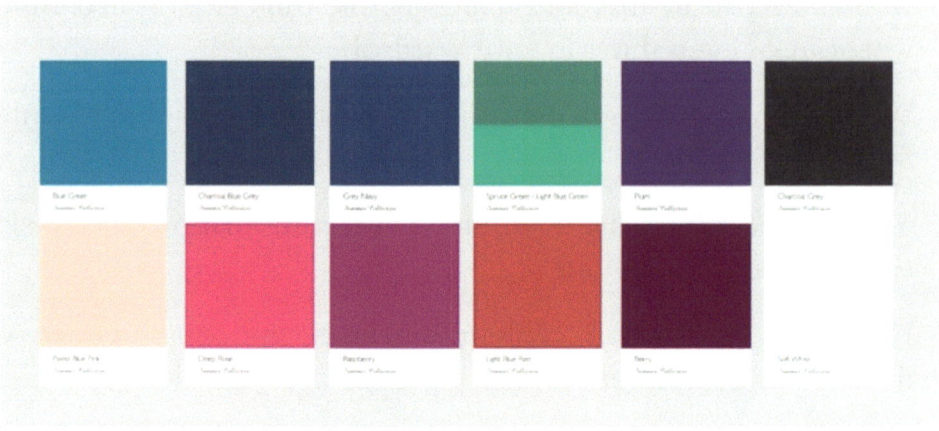

or you can buy them on this totally unique key ring.

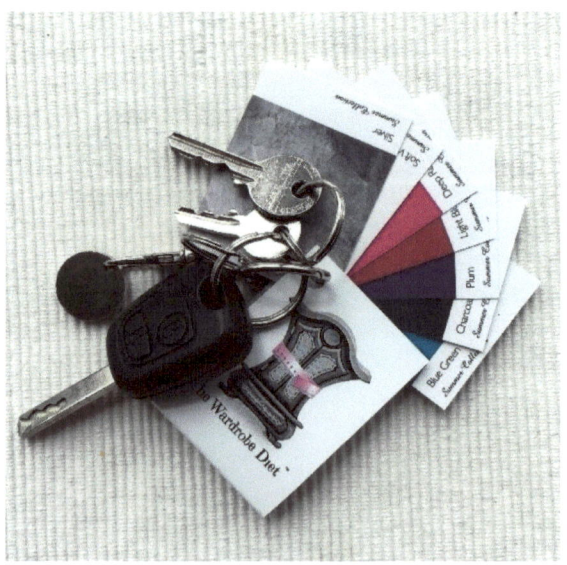

What Step 2 - Your Beautiful Body Shape entails

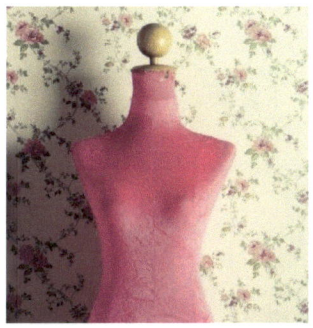

What styles suit you and why certain styles and details will work or not.

Everyone is a different body shape.

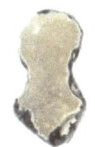 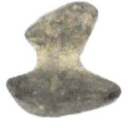 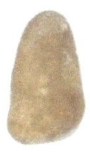 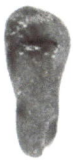 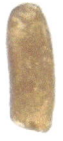 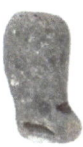

These are my pebble body shapes I use to demonstrate the different shapes (all found on West Worthing beach when I was on my early morning runs).

It started when we were born, and as we grow we are still all different shapes and sizes, and will be all our lives.
These babies are the same age. As you can see, they are completely different shapes, sizes and weights.

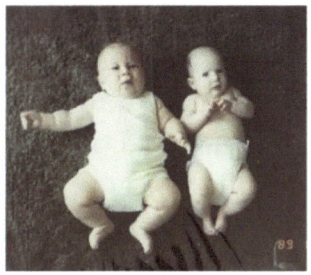

Here's a photo of my sports day. I'm third in from left - grinning like crazy person! Do you remember when you were at school, your class was a mixture of unique shapes and sizes?

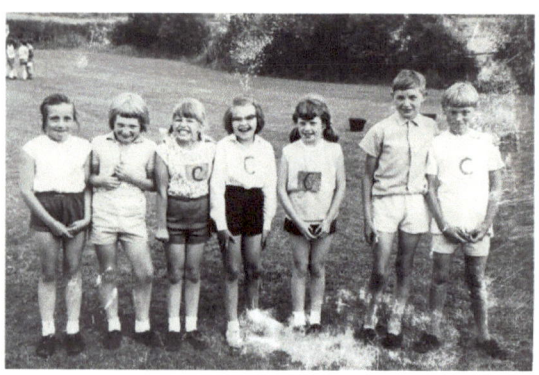

It's your skeleton proportions that determine your body shape; it's not about inches or centimeters. The aim is to create balance using the ideal clothes styles that suit *your* body shape.

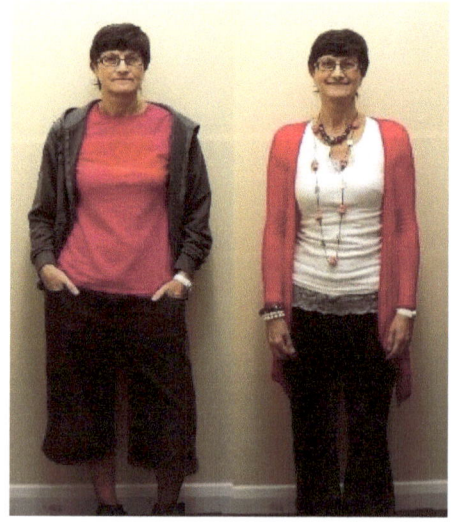

These photos were taken within minutes of each other.
I changed the styles, fit, fabric, colours and added a few style tricks!
She looks great, doesn't she?

As part of our programme you get your personalised styles, either to print off as a pdf (as below)

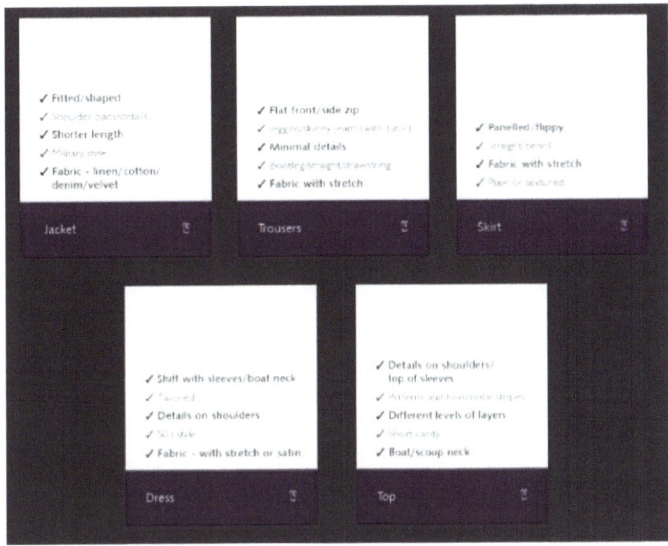

or to buy on this utterly unique key ring.

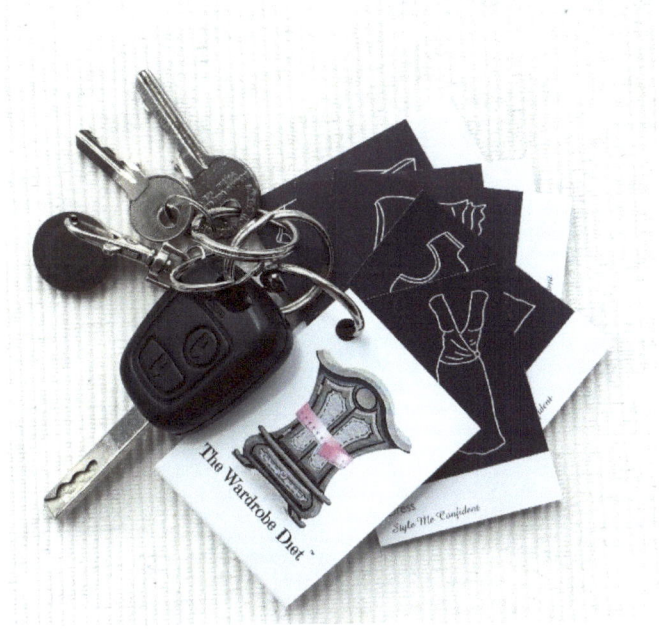

The difference that a choice of fabric can make.

We don't always consider the fabric and sometimes it is this that determines whether an item is flattering or not.
Little thing, big difference.

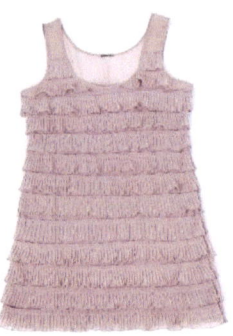

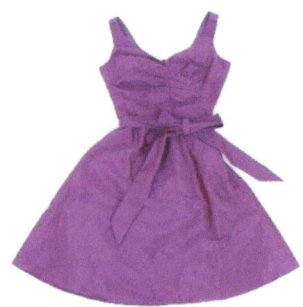

Stretchy fabric   Structured fabric

As a general guideline the curvier you are, the more the fabric needs to have some stretch or 'give' in it.

The more 'straight line' you are, fabrics that are more structured and less stretchy look better on you e.g. cotton, linen, denim.

Most of us are a combination of curvy and straight body lines and so items that are shaped and fitted will suit us.

What Step 3 – Your Wonderful Wardrobe entails

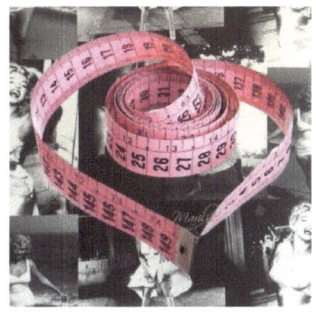

The benefits of an organised wardrobe.

Using your personalised colours and your personalised body shape knowledge, we teach you how to de-clutter and organize your wardrobe so that everything in it is just right for you and your lifestyle.

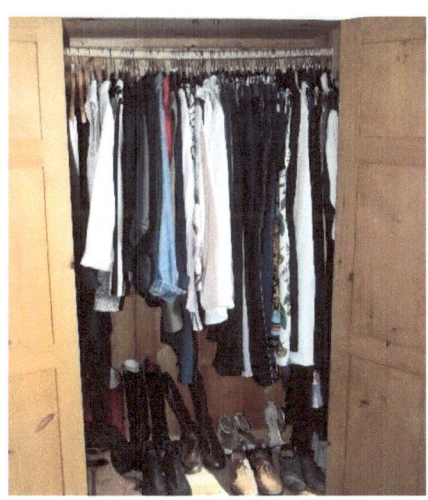

What Step 4 – Your Successful Shopping entails

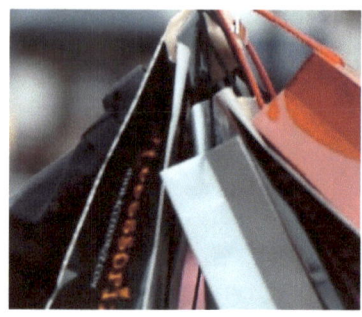

**How to shop successfully to build your
ideal wardrobe of clothes.**

You will have created an essential shopping list from completing the first three steps. This will have key items you need to buy to complete/ update your wardrobe for your lifestyle.

We then teach you the techniques and tricks of shopping successfully so you can build a wonderful collection of clothes that make you happy every time you get dressed.

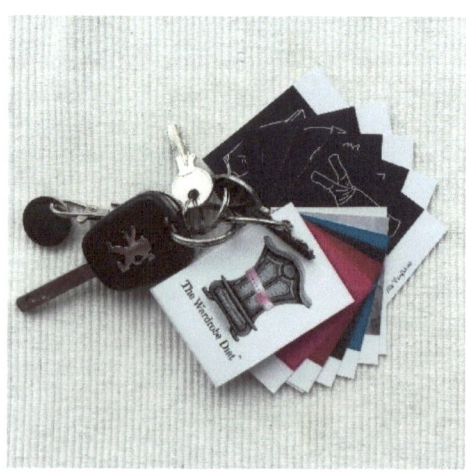

Chapter 3:
Common mistakes and misconceptions

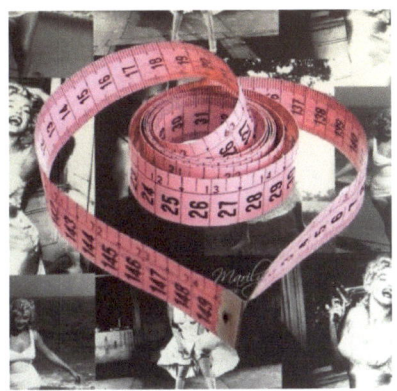

'I had clothes in my wardrobe which were 'orphans' (nothing to go with them) and was at a loss how to wear stuff.

I wore the same styles all the time and felt very boring and frumpy! Now I have learnt new ways to wear the clothes I already had – a complete revelation!'

Jo, Yummy Mummy, Brighton

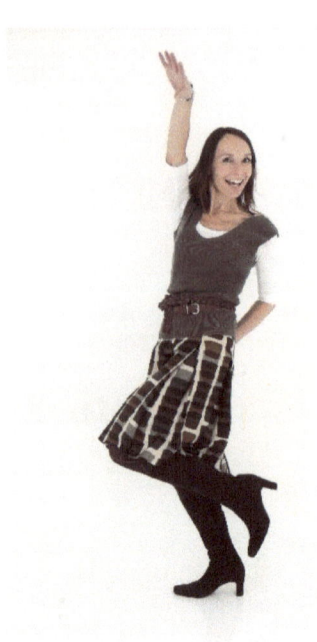

As we said at the beginning, we all have to dress everyday and no-one has ever taught us how !

So understandably we are all likely to make mistakes. Don't worry !

As you are reading this book, you are already on your way to sorting them all out very soon.

As women, we have been plagued with misconceptions fed us from when we were very young...lets kick them into touch with a high heeled shoe!

7 Common Wardrobe Mistakes:

1. multiple items that are the same style;

2. random items that don't go with anything;

3. keep things for 'best';

4. same item in different colours;

5. keep 'sets' together;

6. sizes that don't fit you;

7. too many items squashed in the wardrobe.

4 Common Shopping Mistakes:

1. don't know your flattering colours/styles;

2. get overwhelmed, give up and go home;

3. always go to the same shops;

4. make panic purchases.

Common Body Shape Misconceptions:

You have to be tall and skinny to be sexy and attractive.

Generally, the world we live in today has an incredibly narrow view of what is beautiful - promoted by the extremely biased press, fashion industry and social media.

Believing that we need to look like celebrities/models in magazines/TV is such a waste of time, and energy.

When we are born we are all utterly unique, therefore we cannot possibly all be the same. There is not just one form of beauty and as the saying goes, beauty is in the eye of the beholder.

Let's choose to have the confidence of **not** worrying about our body shape and feeling happy. Confidence is more attractive than anything else you put on your body.

My body shape is 'wrong' — clothes don't fit me like they do on the mannequin.

The mannequins are all the same size, always. Take a peep behind the mannequins, the clothes are frequently pinned, so they always look good.

Please remember - it's never your body that is 'wrong' – it's always the clothes that are 'wrong' for your body, if they don't look good.

Your body shape is yours and we teach you to select the styles that will suit your shape so that you feel confident.

Common Sizing Misconceptions:

Size really doesn't matter – it's only a number – 8, 10, 12, 14, 16, 18, 20, 22, 24, 26, 28, 30…

These numbers really don't mean anything - it's not inches or centimetres or age or number of items we have exhaustedly tried on.

I bet in your wardrobe you have items that are a range of sizes. The size *so* doesn't matter, the *fit* so does.

It's just a guide as to which one to try on. If you try on several of 'the same size' they will all vary in fit.   The size label is just a guide.

You *know* your size will vary from shop to shop, brand to brand, country to country.

You *know* this. You *do*!

No-one *ever* asks you 'what size is that?' They will say 'Wow - that looks great' or 'Where did you get that fabulous…?'

You look bigger if you squeeze into a smaller size, and look slimmer if you choose a size that fits.

While you are adjusting from a lifetime of indoctrination of 'worrying about the size', why not cut the label out and concentrate on looking comfortable and feeling confident.

The fact is that we **all** generally wear 20% of our wardrobe 80% of the time, so we do have a vast amount of clothes that we aren't wearing and so have wasted our hard earned money, valuable time and sometimes much heartache.

Let's see where you are currently and do 'Your Wardrobe Audit'

- You will need a pen and a calculator.

- Allow at least an hour, possibly two, depending on how many wardrobes you have.

- Try not to cheat! Just round up prices of items and be as truthful as possible.

- When you have completed the chart, you may feel horrified, shocked or dismayed at the amount at the end, but please don't beat yourself up…. you can resolve the problem, you are already on your way as you are reading this book!

The Wardrobe Diet: The Wardrobe Audit Chart

My Wardrobe Audit	Jackets	Tops	Jumpers	Trousers	Dresses	Skirts
How many?						
How much money have you spent? (approximately per item) A						
How many _DON'T_ you actually wear? (be honest!) B						
How much have you spent unnecessarily on unworn clothes? A x B	£ +	£ +	£ +	£ +	£ +	£ +

Making a total of £ ....

Just imagine what you could have spent this 'wasted' money on ...holiday?

House improvement? That expensive bag/ shoes? Or an expert to show you how to shop so your wardrobe has no wastage and you have an amazing wardrobe collection just perfect for you..i.e The Wardrobe Diet Programme.....

The Wardrobe Diet ˜

Chapter 4:
Breaking the vicious circle

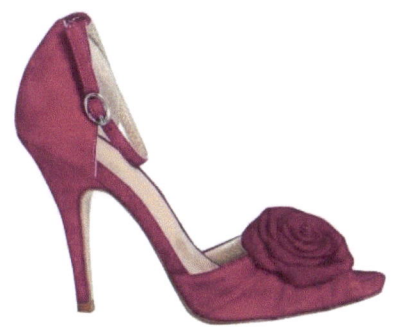

'I thought I had been dressing well and couldn't understand why I felt so negative about myself. You helped me to understand my body shape and showed me clothing tricks that transformed my appearance before my eyes.'

Sarah, 42, professional modern Supermum, Worthing

Put your hand up if you are ready to stop …

- disliking parts of your body, because they make you feel really self-conscious;

- feeling miserable and dissatisfied with what's in your wardrobe and how it makes you feel;

- feeling fed up with always wearing the same sort of clothes;

- keeping far too many clothes ;

- getting frustrated or depressed by clothes shopping as you can't find what you like or what fits;

- wearing what you wore the day before and keeping nice clothes for best;

- putting everybody else first.

Firstly, you need to decide on the size you are happy with. The Wardrobe Diet concept isn't about losing weight (that's not our area of expertise) - it's about empowering you to stay the size you want to be. It is the size you feel comfortable in, can relatively easily maintain. It is ideally a healthy size for your height and frame. You can check out your 'ideal' size on the chart on the next page, though I would go with your instinct to know what feels healthiest for you. And always check with your doctor if you have any health issues to consider.

Whatever size you choose then you eat and exercise to maintain this size. You use your collection of clothes to motivate you to do this.

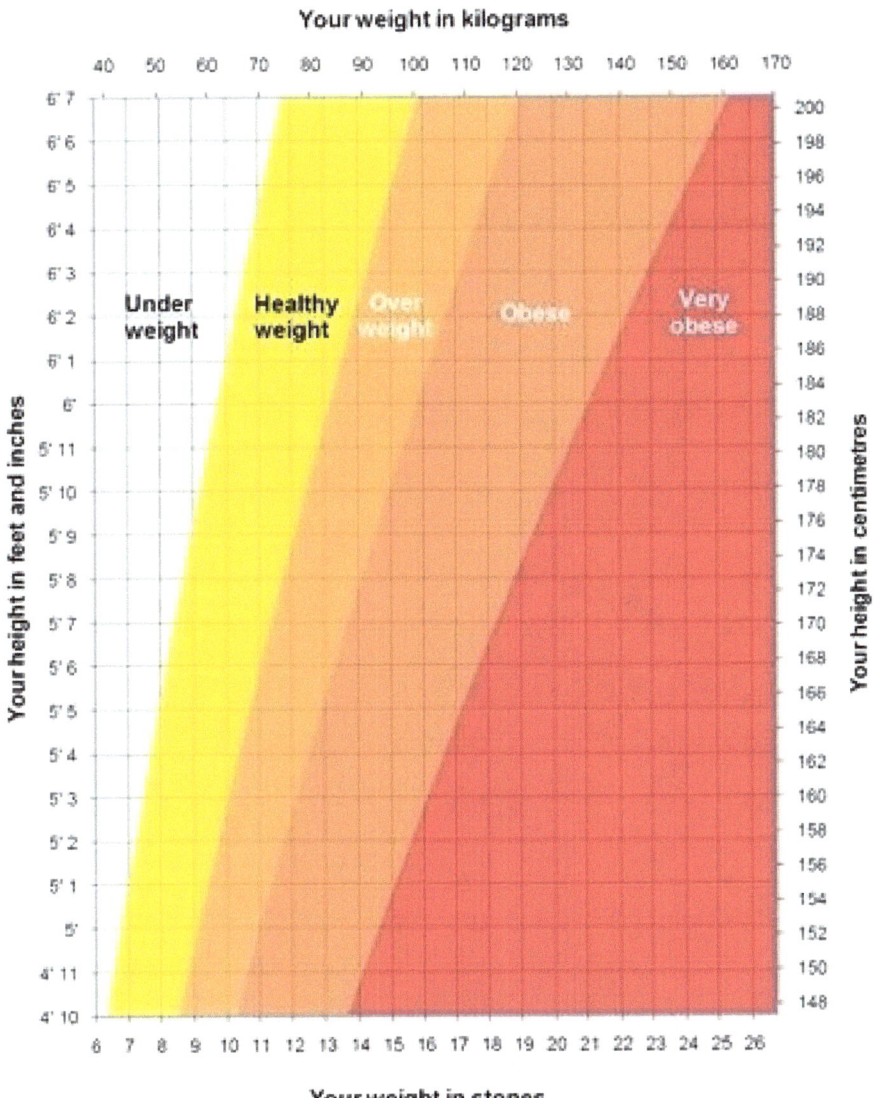

Exercise

Work out what exercise you like the best, is fun, and is easiest to fit into your lifestyle. It's good for us to do some exercise, even if we don't like it, to maintain a healthy body and produce endorphins that are good for our mental health. Regularity is the key.

There is a wealth of choice when it comes to exercise - jogging, running, tennis, golf, walking etc. It could also be a HIIT (high intensity interval training) or Wii-fit session.

If it helps, stick on your headphones and your favourite tunes and go for it!

Yoga and Pilates are great for stretching the body, and are known for improving flexibility and core strength and have been said to improve youthfulness.

Please remember...

Some form of weight-bearing exercise is ideal to prevent osteoporosis later in life, especially for us women. Weight bearing exercises include dancing, running, high impact aerobics, hiking and stair climbing - now that's an easy one to fit in!

As with any change in lifestyle, diet or exercise, you may want to check with your doctor/physician as to the suitability for you.

And remember we are putting ourselves first, so we can 'show up' healthy, happy and smiling for everyone in our lives.

Eating

My favourite saying from my Mum (whose advice was always brilliant), whenever we asked 'Is it fattening?', she would say 'Only if you eat too much of it' – brilliantly simple and so true, and just a bit annoying if it was chocolate or ice-cream!

Sling the scales

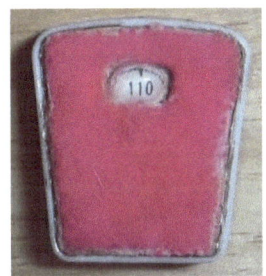 I avoid using the scales in the house as the results are usually disheartening, wildly different from one day to the next and it seems just pointless to me.

I choose to only use scales to weigh my case when I go on holiday – scales are absolutely brilliant for that!

Use your clothes as your 'scales'.

In my experience here are some general healthy top tips to consider to maintain a healthy body:

- drink water every day (sometimes hunger masquerades as thirst so try drinking something when you first feel hungry, if it's not meal time);

- eat three well balanced meals a day, with mini healthy snacks if needed;

- eat fresh food – your five or more a day;

- minimise packet and tinned food;

- infrequent takeaways;

- have little treats so you don't feel deprived;

- tea and Coffee – have the best quality and not excessive;

- limited alcohol - try a smaller glass;

- don't buy bad stuff if you can't help eating it e.g. biscuits, crisps, cheese etc. get your family to support you as it helps them as well. (I've found if you can wait 20-30 minutes then the craving goes away.) We know there is usually no nutrition value in that 'naughty' stuff;

- laughter is the best medicine, have fun and *smile*.

It's about maintaining the same size, so that you can still have cake, or anything else you enjoy - crisps, cheese, wine - but in moderation, so your clothes will always fit.

Today there are many online courses about exercise and nutrition, which can be done easily in the home.

You have to make a judgement for yourself. Every 'body' is different so listen to your body, look after it the best you can and you will gain the benefits of a 'vehicle' in tip top condition.

Chapter 5:
The Wardrobe Diet
What's in it for you?

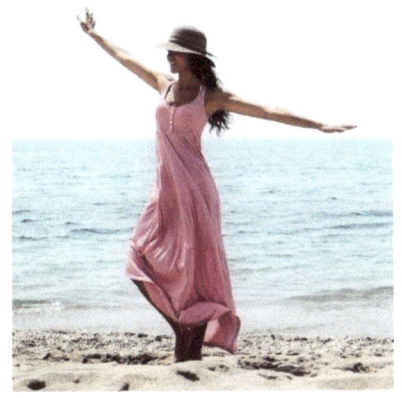

'I just wanted to say thank you SO much. I walked into work with a spring in my step, feeling more confident and happy AND had two compliments on my new outfit - thank you! xxx'

Christina, 30+, retired Olympic Sailor and now

business owner with a young family

We can all do with a boost to our self-esteem and body confidence, which in turn helps us become more assertive and confident in whatever role we play in life.

One of the easiest, most cost effective ways is to adapt what we are wearing. After all we do have to get dressed every day!

Because you have this book you already qualify for our super duper offer of a whopping 30% discount off The Wardrobe Diet Progamme......but hey don't take my word for it - here's what some of my lovely clients have to say.......

'I went into shops and wandered aimlessly, not knowing what to wear. Invariably picked up things that I liked but didn't suit me so when I tried them on, they looked awful – I'd feel very despondent, and so give up.

Now I know exactly what I'm looking for and can disregard things that I like but know don't suit me, so I don't have to go through the negativity of trying things on and feeling bad. Now I'm starting to enjoy shopping and have more positive, successful experiences.'

Marion, modern-day professional, Ashington.

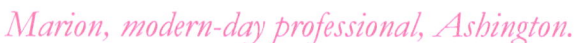

'I love working with Gay because she doesn't 'see' what you 'see' - you know, the bits that your eyes are relentlessly drawn to when you look in the mirror, which is both refreshing and encouraging and she is 'top bird' for pulling pieces together for different occasions.'

Sally, happily retired Mum, Burgess Hill

'Whilst I had been hiding behind black (or navy if feeling adventurous) and choosing colours that I liked not that suited, Gay showed me MY colours, those that enhanced me and my colouring. It sounds over the top to say it changed my life, but it really did.

When I wore my good colors the reaction amongst family and friends was huge. I was getting compliments from strangers!!' *Jo, hospitality professional, Worthing*

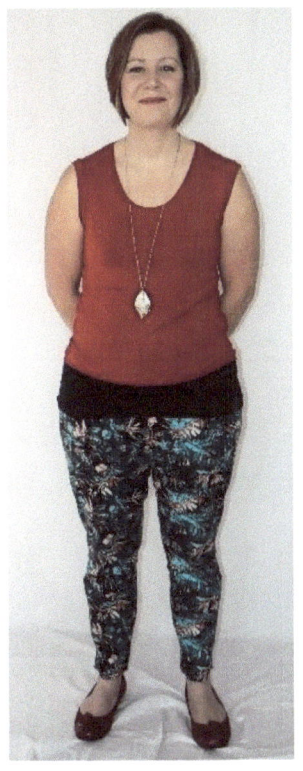
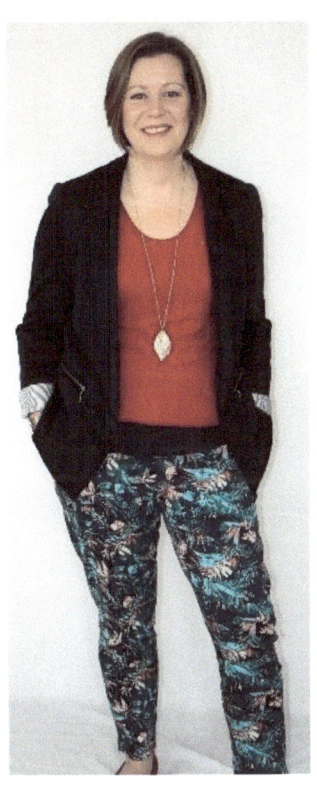

Jo is a triangle body shape. By adding the jacket to her outfit she balances up her shoulders and hips and looks evenly proportioned.

'Working with Gay really helped me get out of the rut of wearing the same old thing, the same old way. She opened up a whole new style world for me and I now experiment with wearing my clothes in different ways and feel stylish but age appropriate. Best of all, I have more time and energy to do other things!'

Fiona, Nifty Fifty, business owner and Mum

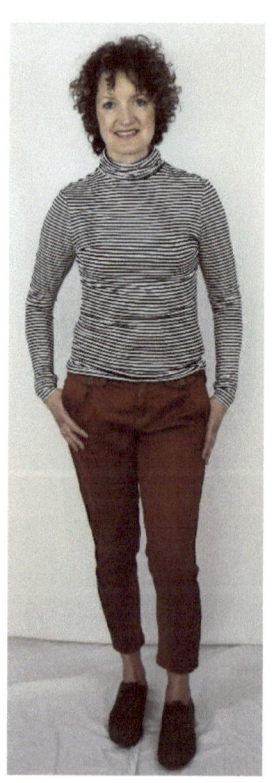 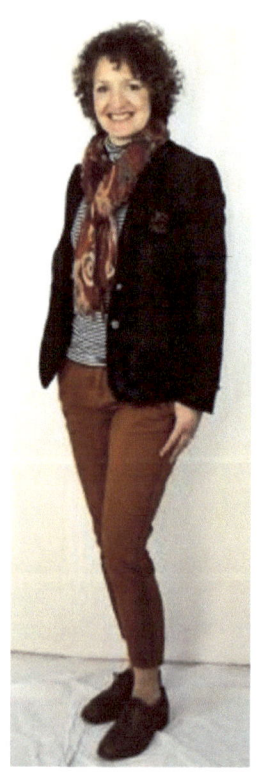

Fiona is a lean column body shape. We chose patterns – the T-shirt and scarf, and different fabrics with textures - cotton, jersey, wool - to achieve this look.

'Since working with Gay, I can honestly say that I am the most confident in my own skin. Through her help and advice, I now know what styles of clothes suit and flatter me, which colours are my best and how to accessorize. Gay is friendly and approachable and always makes me smile with her enthusiasm and kind words.'

Emma, recently married, modern-day Superwoman

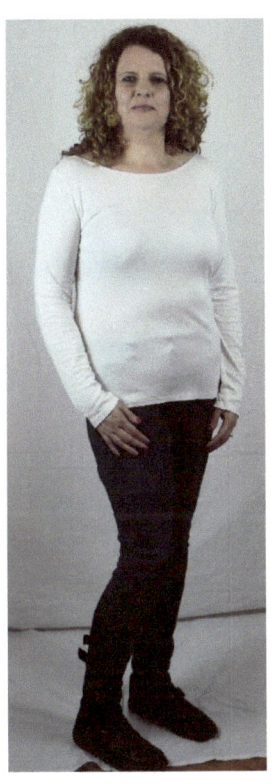 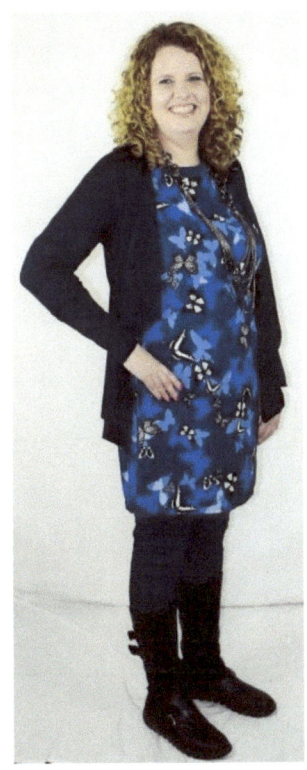

Emma has a rectangular body shape. We used a patterned tunic to 'disguise' any extra tummy weight and an asymmetrical unstructured cardigan to create the illusion of curves. The skinny jeans show off her slim legs.

'I decided I needed help when I was going back to work after my second child was born. I just wore loose baggy trousers, huge tops and always looked scruffy. So on recommendation I saw Gay for some styling and colour and how to turn into a smarter working mum. The results have been amazing. I've received so many compliments that my self-esteem has been boosted hugely and it's all down to Gay's magic.'

Ann, modern-day Supermum and business owner, Emsworth

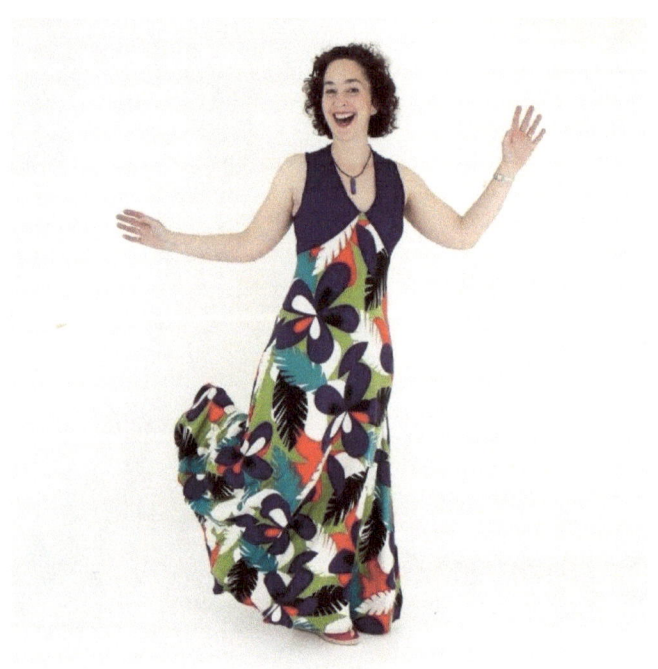

In summary you will:

- be happy that you have a collection of clothes that makes getting dressed a pleasure again;

- be delighted to be wearing everything in your wardrobe;

- your clothes will fit and flatter, making you look and feel super confident;

- wear a selection of colours that make you look healthy and radiant;

- feel relaxed that you always have an outfit, whatever the occasion;

- look modern and up-to-date;

- receive compliments – remember to smile and say thank you;

- save money - no unworn or 'worn once' mistakes and fashion disasters;

- have invested time and money in developing your wardrobe and so have a compelling reason to stay the same size;

- know you are helping the environment by not wasting money on unnecessary purchases.

'I feel a million dollars every time I walk out the door whatever I am wearing and I get compliments all the time. I wish I'd done this years ago'

Maureen, 70+ semi-retired nurse and Grandma

Chapter 6:
Now it's *your* Cinderella moment

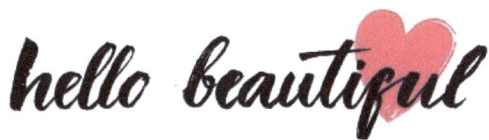

'Not a day goes by when I don't send happy thankful wishes to you and I pat myself on the back for asking for your help.'

Emma, 30, Mum of three, Brighton

We all know the story – Cinderella was treated cruelly by her Wicked Stepmother and made to live in the cellar, do all the chores and be a slave to her step sisters.

Because her loving Mum had taught her to be kind and courageous, she stayed in the background and put everyone else first. She then blossomed when her Fairy Godmother changed her clothes and made her feel a million dollars.

You don't need to be invited to a ball to start your transformation but often there is an event or a situation that becomes your 'Cinderella' moment – it might be becoming a parent, the approach of a big birthday, a new relationship, a new job, the start of a new chapter.

Imagine how much more confident you would feel about yourself, knowing that everything in your wardrobe is a perfect fit for you and your lifestyle?

The Wardrobe Diet will give you your chance to "go to the ball" feeling amazing, just like Cinderella.

Here are a few questions you might want answering:

How much time will each step take me?

Anything from 30 mins to 2 hours

What does it cost?

Usually £190. For you £127

How do I sign up?

Go to **www.thewardrobediet.co.uk** and use the drop down button for code TWD30 to get an exclusive 30% off, as a thank you for buying this book.

Can I pay by card?

Yes, you can use any credit or debit card via PayPal.

Can I follow you on social media?

You can – go to the website www.thewardrobediet.co.uk and click on the links to follow us on Facebook, YouTube, and Instagram.

How do I contact you?

Via email: **gay@thewardrobediet.co.uk**

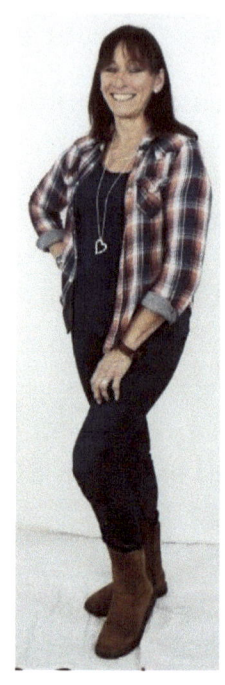

'What The Wardrobe Diet did for me - it simply helped me be happy with my body shape and buy clothes to suit it... and then keep that shape, and all those clothes!! I had a pile of beautiful size 10 clothes – I had 'dieted' to achieve a figure that I thought I loved – and bought clothes to fit it.

Then my weight crept up – so I ended up with clothes in sizes 10, 12 and 14. I was not happy being size 14, so those clothes have now all gone – along with a few pounds.

With size 12 there is some flab, but not too much, and there are curves, instead of stick thin. And I am happier – and can eat and drink without fretting.

But, as the clothes tighten, I follow The Wardrobe Diet™! And because all my clothes fit, I know that I can wear everything in my wardrobe. I love my 'Wardrobe Diet'.'

Kay, just 60, wife and Mum, West Worthing

We are so looking forward to hearing from you.

The Wardrobe Diet Pledge

I will keep to The Wardrobe Diet principles because I know that it motivates me to maintain the size I want to be, which will keep me healthier, fitter and feeling confident.

I will love the body I have been blessed with and aim to be content with it.

I know this "diet" makes me a happier person to live with and has a positive effect on my family and friends.

I know that this "diet" contributes towards the planets environment and is eco-friendly.

I will always be kind, truthful, supportive and encouraging whenever my friends ask for advice and help.

I know that it will help others too, so I will tell them my experience on The Wardrobe Diet.

And so it is….

Signed :

Date :

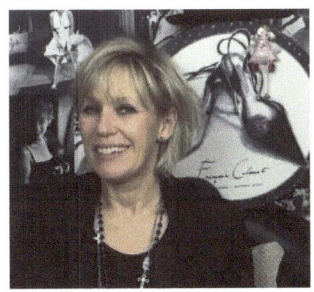

Acknowledgments

Firstly, I would like to thank all my clients, who have given me the momentum to create The Wardrobe Diet™ so that I can help more women all over the world.

Thank you to my business partner Kate, daughters Jessie and Paris, my partner Mark, my dearest twin sister Nan, beloved Ant Bet and my lifelong friends Lynne, Donna, Jacqui, Barbara, Rose and Kay. Your endless support and love has been invaluable and I'll be forever grateful.

And then there's you!

Thank you for reading this book and I hope benefiting from it, as that is my sole reason for doing this.

Bless you. xxx